# THERE IS A RAINBOW IN MY LUNCHBOX

# THERE IS A RAINBOW
# IN MY LUNCHBOX

BY HAYLEY DAVIS, RD

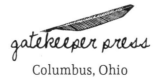

gatekeeper press

Columbus, Ohio

There Is a Rainbow in My Lunchbox

Published by Gatekeeper Press
2167 Stringtown Rd, Suite 109
Columbus, OH 43123-2989
www.GatekeeperPress.com

Library of Congress Control Number: 2022936891

ISBN (hardcover): 9781662926662
ISBN (paperback): 9781662927560
eISBN: 9781662927577

*Dedicated to my loves, Josh and Reece.*
*Endless gratitude to my two favorite taste testers who bring so much color to this world. Thank you for teaching me to always find the rainbow amongst the chaos.*
*I love you both SO much.*

It was lunchtime at school,
my favorite part of the day.

Except this day was different,
in a very colorful way.

# I OPENED MY LUNCHBOX
# TO SEE WHAT WAS INSIDE…

And a beautiful sight caught my eye!

Feeling full of excitement to quickly dig in,
I took one bite, *yum*!

# NOW, LET'S BEGIN…

"CRUNCH"
from the apples,
peppers, and pears.

"MUNCH"
from the strawberries
that were also in there.

NOW, WHAT COLOR
DO THESE FOODS ALL SHARE?

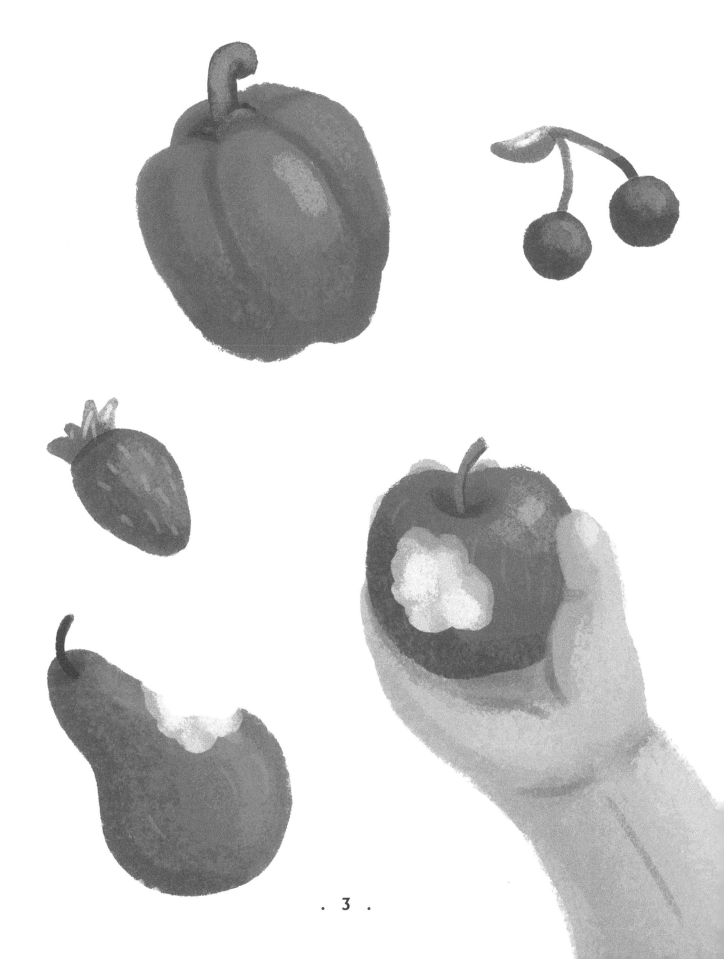

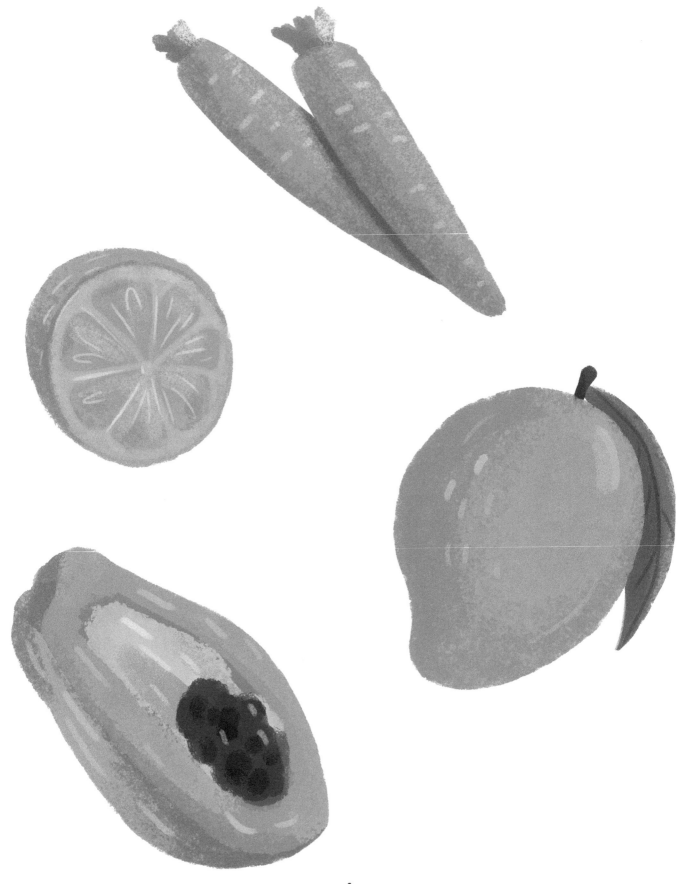

"SLURP"
from the juicy mangoes
and papayas too.

Followed by,
"CHOMP"
from the carrots; oh how my
appetite still grew.

This vibrant color shares
a name with a fruit,
how deliciously unique!

# DO YOU KNOW WHAT COLOR
# WE ARE TRYING TO SEEK?

# SWEETNESS
from the banana slices shaped
like half-moons.

# SOUR

tasting pineapples, now let me
grab my spoon!

All of these colorful flavors
are such a delight.

I'll give you a hint
for this color...

# IT'S QUITE BRIGHT.

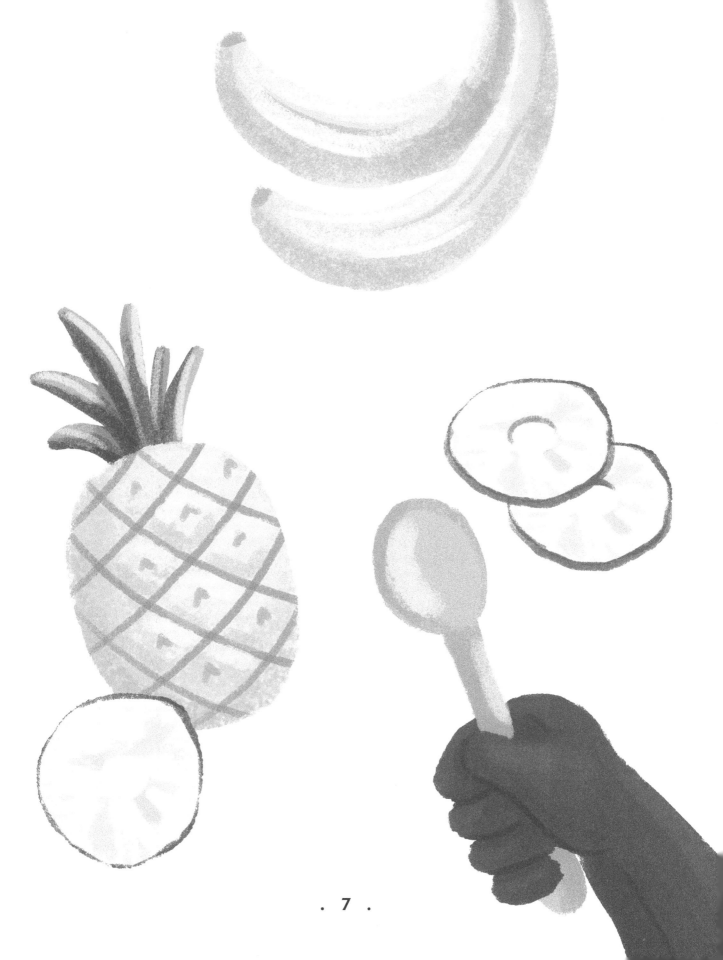

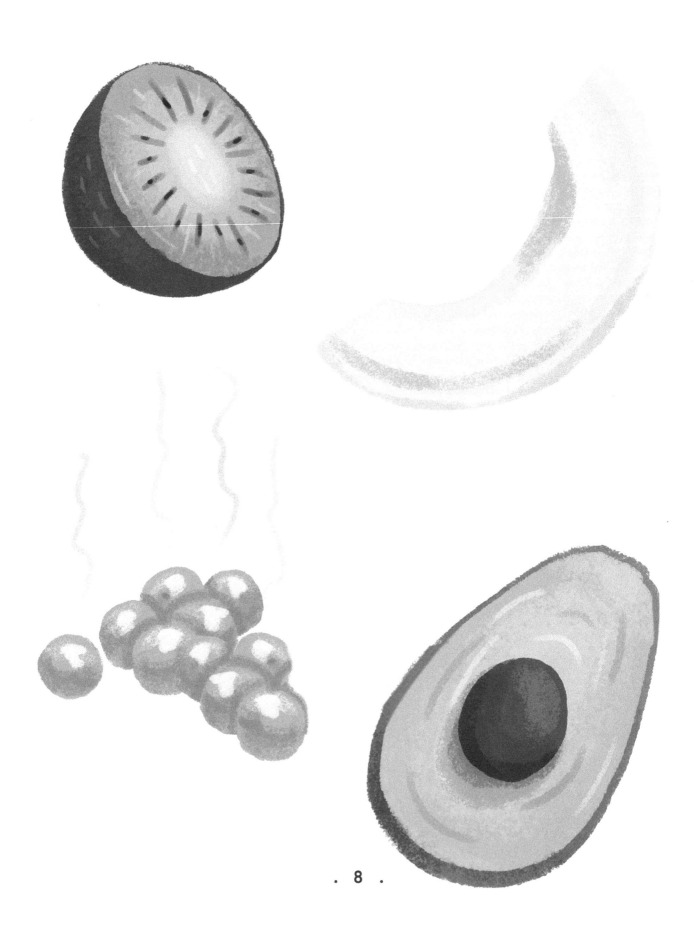

CREAMY
avocados along with
steamed peas.

JUICY

honeydew and
even kiwis!

When eating these foods,
WHAT COLOR OF THE RAINBOW
DO YOU SEE?

The last colorful bites
in my lunchbox are
PURPLE AND BLUE.

Plums, berries, and beets,
just to name a few.

I love tasting all of the colors
from the rainbow.

And eating all of these
colors will help me
GROW, GROW GROW!

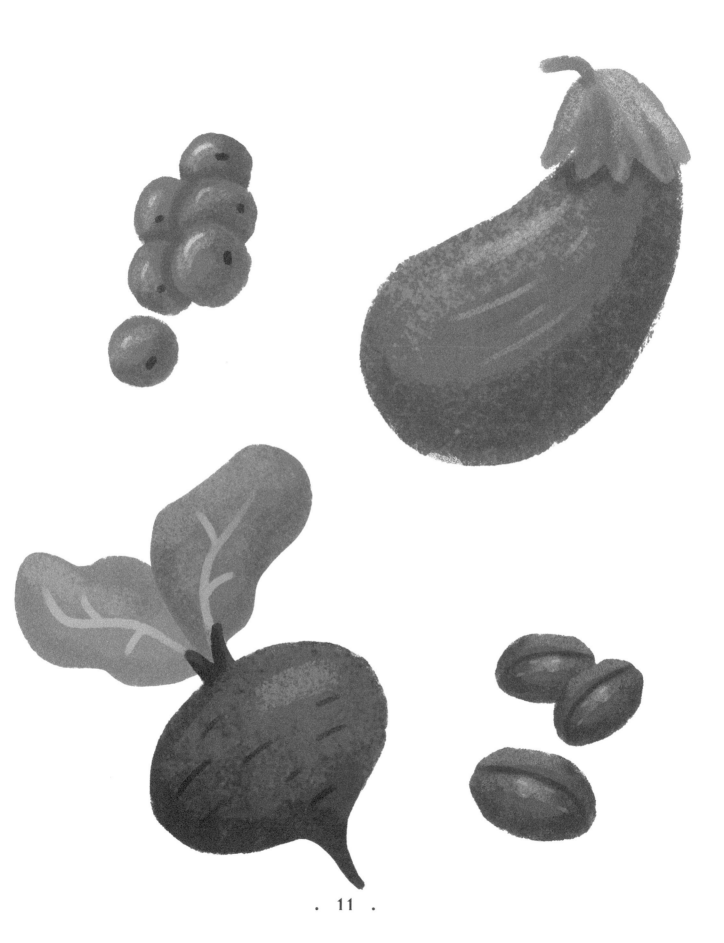

# KEEP TRACK OF THE COLORS YOU EAT EVERYDAY

|  | RED | ORANGE |
|---|---|---|
| **Monday** | | |
| **Tuesday** | | |
| **Wednesday** | | |
| **Thursday** | | |
| **Friday** | | |
| **Saturday** | | |
| **Sunday** | | |

| YELLOW | GREEN | BLUE/PURPLE |
|--------|-------|-------------|
|        |       |             |
|        |       |             |
|        |       |             |
|        |       |             |
|        |       |             |
|        |       |             |

# LET'S LEARN THE HEALTH BENEFITS
# OF EATING THE RAINBOW

Red colored fruits and vegetables help keep our heart healthy by providing our bodies with antioxidants. Antioxidants are made up of vitamins and other nutrients and act as the body's superheroes to get rid of toxins, which act as the body's bad guys that can make us feel sick.

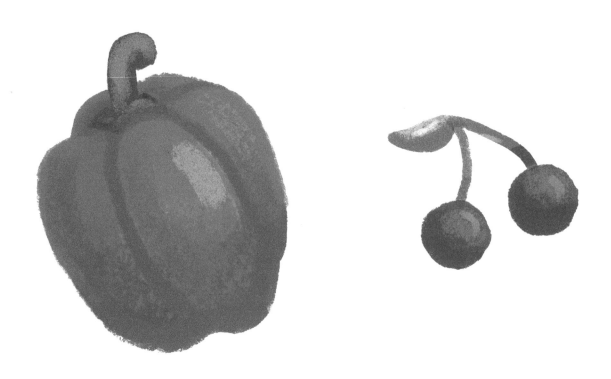

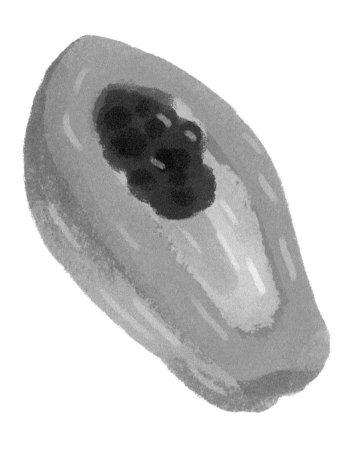

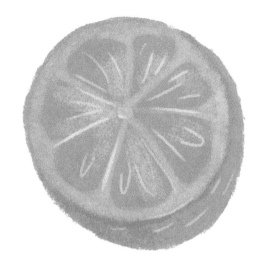

Orange colored fruits and vegetables are packed with vitamin C and vitamin A. Vitamin C is a very important nutrient for our bodies' ability to boost our health and reduce our risk from viral infections, keeping us out of the doctor's office! Vitamin C also helps with our cuts and scrapes if we fall and get hurt; this is the vitamin that helps our boo-boo's heal properly. Vitamin A is also important to keep us healthy and its main job is to support our eyes so we can see well.

Yellow colored fruits and vegetables contain a mineral called potassium. Potassium helps our bodies maintain fluid balance to keep us hydrated and healthy. It also allows our muscles to move and act the way they do. For example, when the doctor taps your knee at your check-up, you will notice your lower leg kicks forward, which is known as a reflex. Potassium helps maintain muscular balance controlling our reflexes.

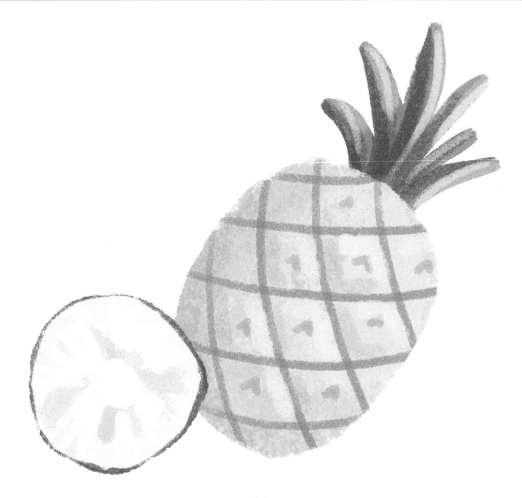

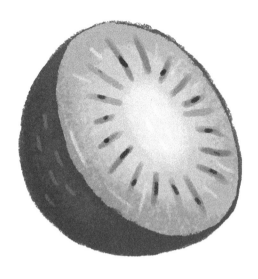

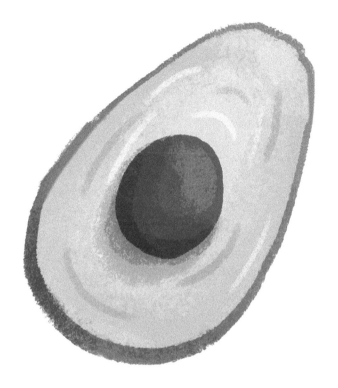

Green colored fruits and vegetables boost our fiber needs to promote healthy digestion. When you eat, your food goes into your tummy and with fiber's assistance it can digest well and leave your body as a cycle. Green fruits and vegetables are full of vitamins and minerals that provide many health benefits. One in particular is calcium which keeps our bones healthy and strong.

Blue/Purple colored fruits and vegetables encourage brain health to keep our memory sharp. This group is what we can thank when we come up with good ideas, or when we remember someone's name. It also contains the body's superheroes known as antioxidants to keep us healthy and strong, preventing the "bad guys" that make us sick to enter our body.

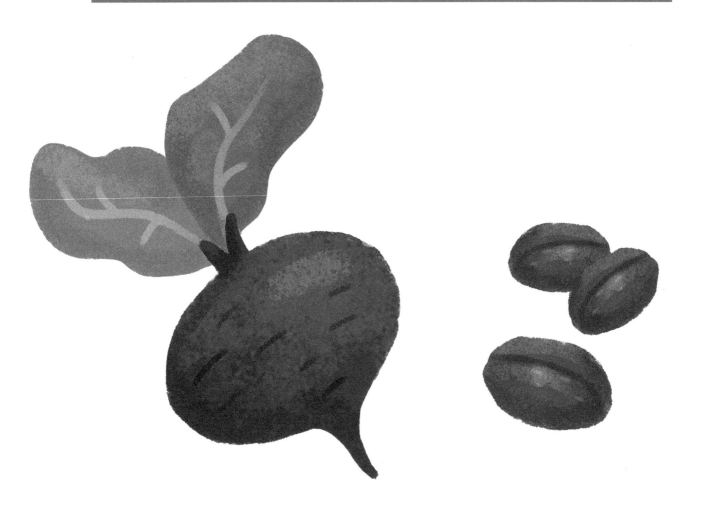

# WHERE DOES "EATING THE RAINBOW" COME FROM?

### On trees:

Apples, oranges, cherries, lemons, mangoes,
peaches, pears, limes, plums

### Above ground:

Pineapples, cucumbers, cabbage, zucchini,
bell peppers, broccoli

### In ground:

Beets, carrots, potatoes, sweet potatoes,
onions, parsnips, ginger

Have you ever seen fruits on a tree or
above the ground in a vine or bush?

If so, can you name them?

Have you ever seen any vegetables
grow in-ground?

If so, can you name them?

# CAN YOU NAME ALL OF THE FRUITS AND VEGETABLES YOU SEE IN THIS RAINBOW?

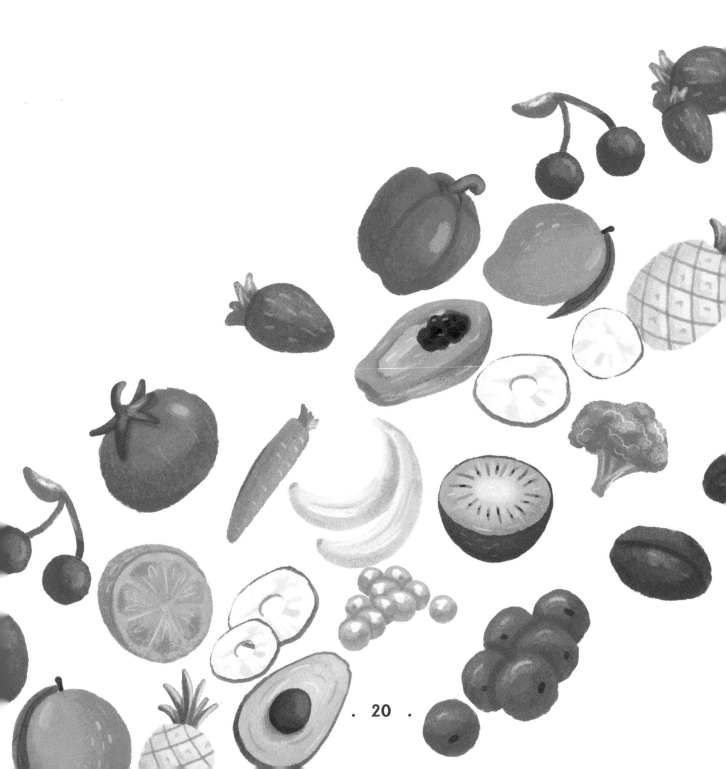

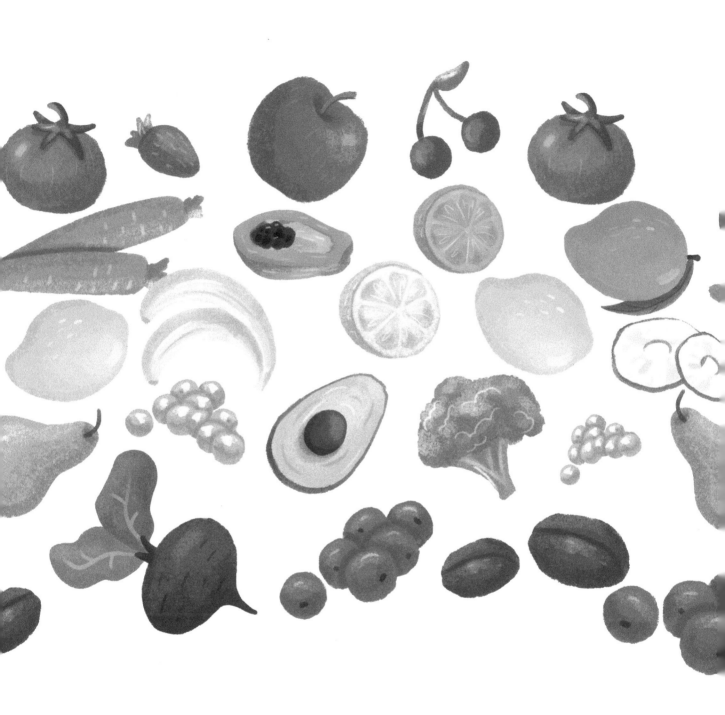

# CAN YOU GUESS WHICH FRUIT OR VEGETABLE IS DESCRIBED BELOW?

I am red. I am crunchy.
I grow on trees.

**What am I?**

I am orange. I boost immunity.
I grow underground.

**What am I?**

I am yellow. I am sweet.
I grow on trees.

**What am I?**

I am green. I look like a mini tree.
I grow above the ground.

**What am I?**

I am blue. I am small.
I grow above the ground.

**What am I?**

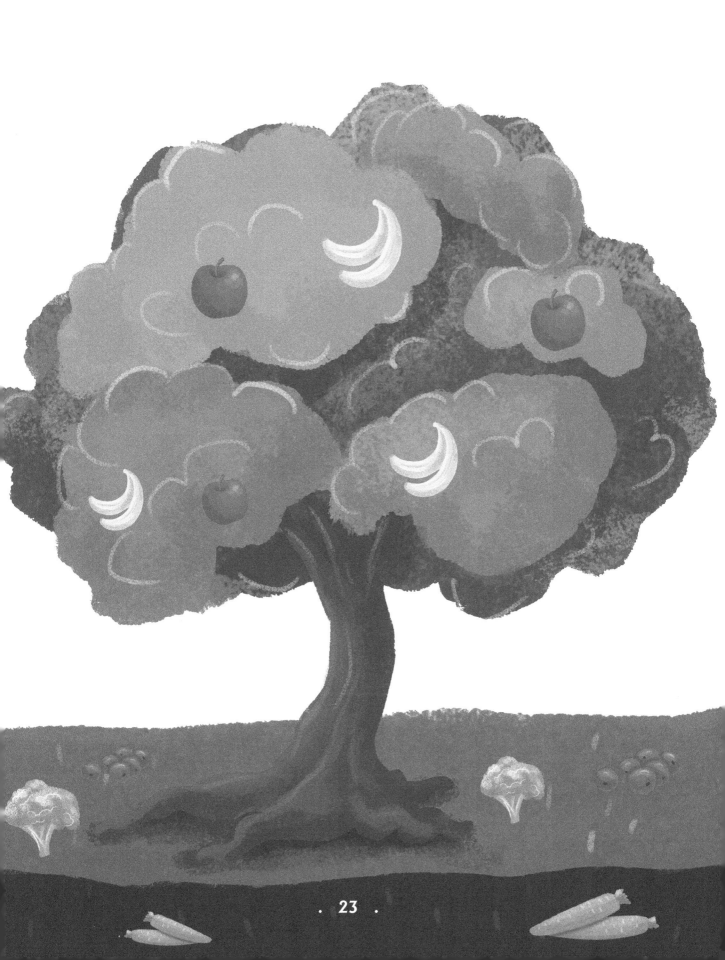

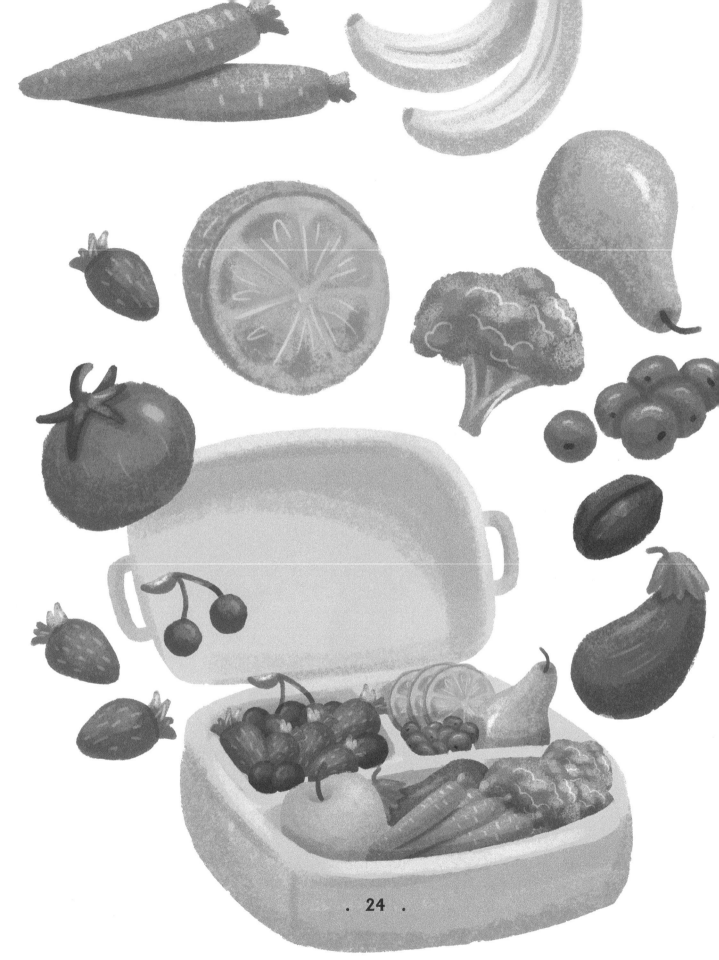

# HAYLEY DAVIS

is a Registered Dietitian, mommy, and wife who loves cooking, eating, and educating people on how to foster a mindful relationship with food. Her desire to become a dietitian stemmed from a love of science and all things nutrition related. She worked in various healthcare settings practicing dietetics. However, the long hours and restrictive environment were not ideal to express her personal creativity within the field of nutrition. She began nutrition consulting, writing for magazines, teaching cooking classes, giving grocery store tours, and educating children on healthy eating.

With her debut children's book, Davis hopes to empower others to adopt healthful eating habits and impress upon children the importance of nutrition and healthy eating. She encourages her family and friends to eat well, prepare their own meals as much as possible, and always aim for a colorful plate.

CPSIA information can be obtained
at www.ICGtesting.com
Printed in the USA
BVHW021947031122
650923BV00002B/27